Low Fiber Diet

6-Week Plan for Restoring

Your Bowel Health

By

Anna Keating

Low Fiber Diet

Copyright © 2017

ISBN: 9781521048313

Warning and Disclaimer

Every effort has been made to make this book as accurate as possible. However, no warranty or fitness is implied. The information provided is on an "as-is" basis. The author and the publisher shall have no liability or responsibility to any person or entity with respect to any loss or damages that arise from the information in this book.

Publisher Contact

Skinny Bottle Publishing

books@skinnybottle.com

Introduction

When the stomach cramps get painful, it is time for concern. Whether you have been diagnosed with a certain bowel condition or you have simply taken it too far with your fried greasy junk food, one thing is certain. Hitting the pause button and taking a break from the heavy foods is the best solution to bring the balance back to your gut. And this book will show you how to do it.

Although the long-term goal of leading a healthy lifestyle is optimal for improving and maintaining bowel health, the low fiber diet is a great first step. However, when the bowels get upset, it is the best cure for restoring abdominal health. If your doctor has suggested cutting back on fiber for some time, then this book is your solution.

From determining if you really are a low fiber candidate, to showing you the path to achieving gut balance, this book will be a real eye-opener to anyone whose bowel health has been compromised. Teaching you the quickest, easiest and least painful way to 'reset' your gut health while gearing you up with a 6-week low fiber meal plan to get you started, this book will help you normalize your bowel function in no time.

Join me on this fiberless ride and let's combat the inflammation together!

The Truth Behind Fiber

'Add more fiber to your diet.' If you have ever had stomach issues, then chances are, you have heard this one before. When constipation pays us a visit, the doctors usually prescribe fiber. The truth is that adding fiber to your diet can bring numerous benefits to your life. Dietary fiber that can be found in whole grains, fruits, legumes, and vegetables, is not only beneficial, but essential for a healthy and balanced diet.

But what exactly is fiber? Fiber is that component of plants that travels through our bowels without first being digested. Dietary fiber can be classified into two categories:

1.   **Soluble Fiber** – This type of fiber is usually found in oats, carrots, citrus, beans, peas, barley, apples, and psyllium. It can dissolve in water and become gelatinous. This gel-like fiber material can keep cholesterol and glucose levels in check.

2.   **Insoluble Fiber** – Insoluble fiber is found in whole wheat flour, nuts, wheat bran, green beans, potatoes, green beans, etc., and it is adds bulk to the stool.

Unlike other key nutrients such as fat or carbohydrates that get easily broken down during the process of digestion, fiber passes intact (and undigested) through the intestines and then out of the body. And while this may seem like an unhealthy thing, the fact that fiber passes through the bowels undigested, is what makes it so important to our health.

Fiber moves the stool through the digestive tract and it is what keeps the colon and bowels in general, healthy. If you still cannot understand how fiber gives bulk to the stool, think of it as a sponge. Just like a sponge, fiber can absorb intestinal fluids and with that, soften the stool, which speeds its way out of your body. It also increases the healthy gut bacteria. Those beneficial little bugs that reside in your gut actually feed off the fiber you consume. This allows them to flourish and produce fatty acids that have incredibly beneficial properties.

But fiber is not only in charge of keeping your gut healthy; it can improve your overall health in many different ways:

- It helps you lose and maintain weight

- It lowers the risk of diabetes

- It reduces the risk of developing some cancers (especially colorectal)

- It has detoxifying properties

- It makes the bones healthier

- It lowers the risk of suffering from a heart disease

If sugar is your health's worst enemy, then fiber is just the opposite. It is a crucial part of your diet that enables your body to function properly. And while this is a common fact today, the importance of fiber was not so well-known a couple of decades ago. It all started in 1971, when the Irish surgeon Dr. Denis Burkitt published his paper on fiber. In that paper, Dr. Burkitt hypothesized the observation he had made while living in Uganda. According to him, the Ugandans produced four times as much waste as did the Americans who lived there, and he strongly believed that it was a result of their high fiber diet. His observations and ideas quickly became accepted and practiced by the Western culture. His book, *Don't Forget Fibre in Your Diet,* became a huge hit, and Dr. Burkitt became known as the 'fiberman' — or the person who solved the mystery.

Many studies have been conducted since Dr. Burkitt's page-turner was published, and all of them confirm the fiberman's theory. Fiber is an important nutrient. But do we all benefit from fiber intake the same way? Unfortunately, no. Although for healthy people, while consuming a diet rich in fiber can only be beneficial, not everyone's digestive tracts function in the same way. For those who have super-sensitive bowels or struggle with certain medical conditions, fiber can actually do more harm than good. Check out the next chapter and find out whether or not you are a candidate for a low-fiber diet.

Stepping Away from the Fiber

If you have just grasped what fiber means and does to your body, then chances are you are now wondering why on earth anyone would go on a low fiber diet. So why would someone need to step away from the fiber if it makes the stool bulkier? Before I delve deeply into explaining when and how to embark on this low fiber train, let me first explain to you why a doctor would choose to purge fiber from your plate.

Sure, the fiber is extremely healthy and beneficial for most people, but not every human body has the same needs all the time. Sometimes, when we take it too far with our unhealthy diet, or when we become suddenly hit by a certain medical condition, our bowels become upset. When our intestinal tract is begging us to give it a break, lowering fiber intake is the only way we can allow our intestines to rest. By reducing fiber, we lower the food waste that has to pass through the intestines, which gives our bowels the chance to take their well-deserved break and heal properly.

But, who needs a low fiber diet? Your doctor may suggest lowering your fiber intake if you have been struggling with some of these conditions:

Crohn's Disease. Crohn's disease is an inflammatory disease of the bowels. It is usually the small intestine that is inflamed, which makes it difficult to digest food and absorb all the important nutrients from it. This causes diarrhea which can be quite severe for some patients. This is quite a challenging disease to treat, as most of the process of digestion occurs in the small intestine.

If you have been diagnosed with Crohn's disease, then chances are your doctor has already put you on a low fiber diet. Why is that important? By avoiding fiber-rich foods, you lessen the pressure on your bowels and make the gas, cramps, bloating, and other related symptoms, much more manageable.

Ulcerative Colitis. Just like Crohn's disease, ulcerative colitis is also a bowel inflammatory disease; however, it is not the small intestine that it is inflamed, but the colon and the large intestine. This disease is known to cause ulcers in the colon, rectum, and large intestine that can be quite painful and can cause diarrhea and bloating during flare-ups. And while there isn't a particular diet that can magically cure a patient with ulcerative colitis, the low fiber diet has proven to be quite successful in reducing the pain, lowering the symptoms, and increasing the time one has between the flare-ups.

Diverticulitis. This painful disease results from inflammation and infection of the diverticula or the small pouches found in the lining of the colon and large intestine. This condition can be very painful, resulting in fever, nausea, and a pretty noticeable change in the movement of the bowels. And while severe diverticulitis may require immediate hospitalization and surgery, those who suffer from mild diverticulitis can treat themselves with antibiotics and a simple change in their diet. It is possible for a diverticulitis patient to be advised to start a liquid diet for a couple of days and then shift to healthy, low fiber foods. This low-fiber diet can help you restore balance to the bowels and relieve the diverticula inflammation.

Gastroparesis. When gastroparesis occurs (which basically means delayed stomach emptying), the low fiber diet is the best cure. When your gastric emptying is delayed, it usually results in symptoms such as reflux, vomiting, abdominal pain, bloating, and nausea. Although patients with severe cases may have to stick to a liquid diet for a while and process all the food in a blender before consumption, the general guidelines for treatment of this condition are the same – eat small meals, slowly and regularly, and decrease fiber intake.

It is important to know that the foods that are rich in fiber only contribute to the delay of the gastric emptying, and therefore, should be avoided.

Bowel Obstruction. A bowel obstruction is any kind of intestine blockage that prevents the food from being digested properly. The symptoms of this blockage are usually abdominal pain, vomiting, nausea, and cramps. And though a simple bowel obstruction may not seem like something as severe as Crohn's disease, it is not uncommon for the patient to end up in surgery. However, most patients suffering from bowel obstruction have managed to clear food passage through the body with bowel rest and a low fiber diet.

Major Abdominal Surgery. If you have to undergo major abdominal surgery, then this is the best book to help you with your post-op recuperation. Whether you have had a C-section or had to have an intestinal blockage surgically removed; after any kind of abdominal surgery, a low fiber diet is an absolute must.

After a surgery, your bowels need some time to get back to their original state, which makes it pretty obvious that they cannot function as well as usual. To allow the intestines to heal properly, it is crucial not to overburden them and force them to work harder than they are able to. That means that in order to reduce the volume of waste that passes through the intestines, you have to lower the amount of fiber you consume. This low-fiber diet can help your bowels heal after a surgery the right way.

Certain Treatments. Some treatments such as chemotherapy or radiation treatments, can also upset your stomach and cause digestion related troubles. If you have been experiencing cramps, abdominal pain, or diarrhea after a certain treatment, then perhaps it is time for you to lower your fiber intake and give your gut a chance to get well. If you consult with your doctor he/she will probably put you on a temporary low fiber diet. If that is the case, then the meal plan in this book it is the best relief for your belly cramps.

Colonoscopy Preparation. Although this is really only for three days or so, if you have to undergo a colonoscopy, the doctors will put you on a low fiber diet a couple days prior the procedure. The meal plan from this book will give you good insight of exactly what should and what shouldn't be put on your plate.

What About Diarrhea?

If you have been struggling with diarrhea only, then you are probably confused. Will increasing or lowering your fiber intake help you relieve the symptoms? If you increase the fiber intake, it can absorb the intestine fluids, increase the frequency of the bowel movements and improve diarrhea. But that is not always the case. There are many instances that when in the case of diarrhea, fiber did nothing but worsen the symptoms. Sometimes a low fiber diet is also the perfect solution for this annoying condition. However, before you decide whether to up your oats and beans consumption or purge them from your diet, I highly suggest you consult with your physician and choose the best approach for diarrhea, according to your unique symptoms. Sometimes, diarrhea may only be a symptom of what is a more complicated bowel condition.

Regardless of the reason your doctor had for putting you on a low fiber diet, the best thing you can do in order to allow your body to heal is to follow the medical advice and give yourself the chance to recuperate.

The Low Fiber Diet

The low fiber diet supports proper foods digestion by lowering the intact materials that passes through the intestines. The low fiber diet is specially designed to decrease the volume, as well as the frequencies of the food waste, so the digestive system can get back to normal.

Like I said, this is a diet that people usually embark on after experiencing bowel-related discomforts. To lessen the aggravating symptoms, one must cut back on the consumption of food that can irritate the bowels. The low fiber diet is rich in such foods and it is the perfect cure for digestive tract disorders.

However, know that not all of us are the same, and just because this diet has helped someone with Crohn's disease lessen their symptoms, it does not necessarily mean that it will do the same for you. But if you are looking for a general solution to these kinds of problems, well, you have found one! The low fiber diet has proven to be extremely successful with people whose bowel health used to be compromised.

The Benefits

Although a diet that is low in fiber is considered unhealthy, when you struggle with any of the conditions mentioned in the previous chapter, or some other intestine discomfort, lowering fiber intake is the only healthy solution to your problem. Although fiber is an extremely healthy nutrient — when the gut is compromised — it can be the bowel's worst enemy. Just imagine what can happen to your bowels if you decide to curb your hunger with a bowl of a bean chili a few days after an abdominal surgery.

This low-fiber diet was specifically formulated and intended only for the sensitive gut, so it can:

-       Improve digestion

- Lessen pain

- Get rid of abdominal cramps

- Give the bowels time to heal

- Reduce inflammation

- Remove intestinal blockage

- Improve one's dietary tolerance

How Does It Work?

First of all, it is of crucial importance to mention that the low fiber diet shouldn't be a lifestyle. It is not a healthy, everyday diet that one should follow on regular basis. The low fiber diet should and must be followed only in the short term. This diet is designed to help people treat their adverse abdominal condition and restore bowel health. Once the inflammation, pain, or intestinal blockage has been alleviated, the patient should gradually start increasing their daily fiber intake.

Although your doctor should be the one making recommendations of exactly how strict of a diet you should follow, the general low fiber diet guidelines are that a person's daily fiber intake shouldn't be more than 10 to 15 grams.

The low fiber diet is quite restrictive and not so nutrient dense. The only risk of the low fiber diet is that it does not meet recommended nutritional needs. If your doctor has prescribed a short-term low fiber diet, then you probably shouldn't have any side effects. However, if you are supposed to follow the low fiber guidelines for a longer period of time, then perhaps it is best to consult with a registered dietitian, who can make sure that your unique nutritional needs will be met, and that your overall health will not suffer.

Low Fiber vs. Low Residue Diet

If you have been advised to follow a low fiber diet, then chances are you have already come across the term 'low residue diet.' And while these two diets are known to be used interchangeably, they actually are two very different things. They may seem like they are the same diet at first, but once you look closely, you may find that the low residue diet is more restrictive.

Both diets limit the fiber intake, except the low residue diet limits dairy products completely and is quite more restrictive when it comes to eating meat. And while the low residue diet can also help people treat bowel conditions, not everyone needs to follow such a stringent regimen. Unless your doctor suggests otherwise, you can safely enjoy a glass of milk with your breakfast.

The low residue diet usually includes less than 7-8 grams of fiber per day, which is not something that every person with compromised gut should follow.

Dos and Don'ts

When it comes to choosing a diet to follow, there really isn't a one-size-fits-all type of solution. Every diet should be tailored according to the person's unique condition in order to meet all of their nutritional needs. The point isn't to give up if you don't experience good results at first, but to mix and match the ingredients allowed so you can find the best possible solution for your condition.

If you experience bloating after you drink a glass of milk, try to limit your dairy intake to a minimum. If you, however, feel that eating broccoli stems may not be irritating to your bowels, feel free to incorporate them into your diet and see what happens. There are patients who can easily digest bananas and kiwis, while apples will give them cramps. There are also those who can safely consume apples, but do not feel that comfortable after eating kiwi. Whatever you do, just make sure to practice moderation. If and when you decide to add some foods that contain a higher amount of fiber back into your diet, it is highly recommended that you consult with your doctor first.

The Low Fiber Plate

If 'what to eat now?' was the first thing that came to your mind when your doctor informed you that you should start a low fiber diet, know that there is no reason for you to feel discouraged. The low fiber diet may be restrictive and prevent you from enjoying a spicy burrito for the time being, but that does not mean that your meals should be pale, tasteless, and boring. Who can suffer on a diet that allows meat, white bread, cakes, and cookies? The low-fiber diet may not be the healthiest long-term solution, but I am absolutely certain that you will not have any food cravings while following this diet.

Grains. Whole grains are packed with fiber and therefore, will certainly cause distress to those whose bowel health is not so great. Instead of choosing the otherwise recommended products, go for the less healthy version and choose white refined products.

Allowed:

- White Bread

- Plain White Pasta

- White Rice

- Crackers

- Cold Cereals

- Refined Hot Cereals (like Cream of Wheat)

- Waffles and Pancakes made from white flour

Not Allowed:

- Brown Rice

- Oats

- Quinoa

- Granola

- Millet

- Whole Wheat Flour

- Whole Wheat Pasta, Whole Wheat Cereals, Whole Wheat Crackers

- Barley

Vegetables. We all know how important vegetables are to our health, and therefore, including them in your low fiber diet is more than essential.

Allowed:

All veggies except the ones mentioned in the 'not allowed' section can be enjoyed on a low fiber diet. Some great choices that contain less than 2 grams of fiber per serving (100 grams) are:

- Cucumbers

- Tomatoes

- Zucchini

- Green Peppers

- Romaine Lettuce

- Carrots

- Mushrooms

- Onions

- Asparagus

Not Allowed:

- Broccoli

- Corn

- Parsnips

- Brussels Sprouts

-      Artichokes

Legumes. Unfortunately, all legumes are high in fiber and should not be included in this diet. Lentils, beans, green beans, okra, and peas, are not allowed.

Fruits. Usually, when a serving of fruit has less than 2.5 grams of fiber, it is considered to be a low fiber fruit.

Allowed:

-      Honeydew

-      Cantaloupe

-      Watermelon

-      Grapes

-      Ripe Bananas

-      Ripe Peaches

-      Ripe Apricots

-      Pineapple

Not Allowed:

-      Berries

-      Figs

-      Prunes

- Dried Fruits

Note that just because a serving of a certain type of fruit provides you with a considerable amount of fiber, a smaller quantity of that type of fruit will not. If a certain type of fruit isn't on the allowed list, that doesn't mean you can never enjoy that yummy and fruity taste you love so much. For instance, just because one cup of cherries can pack you with nearly 3 grams of fiber (2.9 to be exact), that doesn't mean that you are not allowed to taste a cherry while following this diet. If you crave the taste so much, know that five cherries will provide you with less than a gram of fiber.

Dairy. Dairy products such as milk, cheese, yogurt, buttermilk, and sour cream, contain no fiber. However, dairy products are known to cause bowel discomfort, so if you are even slightly lactose intolerant, it is probably best to leave dairy products out of your meal plan. If you don't have problems with lactose, however, feel free to pack your diet with those amazing sources of calcium, protein, and vitamin B12.

Allowed: All normal dairy products

Not Allowed: Dairy products that contain nuts, seeds, and grains. For instance, yogurt with oats.

Protein Foods. Protein is an essential macronutrient that plays the most important part in repairing tissue and producing enzymes and hormones. It is the key nutrient for restoring your bowel health, so make sure not to skip adding some protein to your plate. For those of you who are vegetarian or vegan, things may be a little more challenging. If you don't eat either meat, fish, or eggs, then talk to your doctor and ask him or her to prescribe you some supplements. Adding some protein powder to your shakes is another great way to up the protein intake.

Allowed:

- Well-Cooked Lean Meat (chicken, turkey, lean beef, and lamb)

- Cooked Fish

- Cooked Eggs

Not Allowed:

- Raw Eggs

- Raw Fish

- Raw or Rare Meat

- Fatty Cuts of Meat

- Pork

Fats. Here is more great news for all the fat lovers! Most fats and dressings are allowed on the low fiber diet.

Allowed:

- Butter

- Margarine

- Mild Salad Dressings

- Mayonnaise

- Ketchup

- Mild Mustard

- Vegetable Oils

- Plain Gravies

- Creamy Peanut Butter

- Whipped Cream

<u>Not Allowed:</u>

- Olives

- Avocados

- Seeds

- Nuts

- Poppy Seed Dressing

- Horseradish

- Crunchy Peanut Butter

Miscellaneous. If you thought that you should give up satisfying your sweet tooth for the sake of your bowel health, then you were wrong! Most of the sweet stuff will not upset your gut and is approved for this low fiber diet. However, keep in mind that you have to be moderate and not curb other cravings with tons of sugar.

<u>Allowed:</u>

- Sugar

- Honey

- Jelly

- Seedless Fruit Jam

- Hard Candy

- Plain Cakes

- Plain Cookies

Plain Biscuits

- Pastries

- Pies

- Sherbet

- Frozen Yogurt (if made with allowed ingredients)

- Smooth Puddings

- Jellies

- Rice Puddings

- Ice Cream (if made with allowed ingredients)

- Coffee

- Tea

Not Allowed:

- Any desserts made with coconut, nuts, seeds, dried fruit, chocolate syrup

- Candy with chocolate and nuts

- Cocoa Powder

- Chocolate

- Popcorn

Low Fiber Diet Guidelines

Wait before you decide to drown your steak in butter and put it on your grill. There are a couple of other things that everyone who is about to follow a low fiber diet must be aware of.

The previous chapter explained exactly which ingredients should and shouldn't be a part of the low fiber diet, but not how to consume them. There are some general low fiber guidelines that need to be followed, however, keep in mind that some of them may still upset your bowels. If that is the case, please consult with your physician to pinpoint the problem and include only what will not cause discomfort.

Raw is Off-Limits

When I say raw, I do not only mean raw fish and eggs. Once you embark on the temporary low fiber lifestyle, you will have to say farewell to munching on baby carrots and apples ... at least until you cook them well. Raw foods may burden your intestines and therefore should be avoided. All vegetables must be cooked first (except cucumbers and tomatoes.) Fruits must be also cooked, or consumed canned or pureed. The only fruits that can be consumed raw are ripe bananas, ripe peaches, ripe apricots, and soft melons.

Peel and Deseed before Consumption

All fruits and veggies must be peeled and deseeded first, no matter if you are about to cook them or eat them raw. And yes, that also includes tomatoes and cucumbers. The food that will end up on your plate must be skinless and seedless so your not-yet-healed bowels can process and digest it well.

Cooking Tips

Fried food is absolutely off-limits. Foods that are fried cause cramps and stomach discomfort, which is the last thing that a person with upset bowels would want. The best cooking techniques are those that will keep the food moist, such as boiling, steaming, braising, and stewing. Avoid roasting and grilling the food, as well, as this cooking method can make the food very dry and tough, which will be hard for your gut to digest.

Taking Supplements

Many people believe that they need to take supplements because this low fiber diet lacks many key nutrients. And while there is no doubt that this is not the healthiest diet to follow, it can still provide essential nutrients. When your bowels are inflamed, you end up absorbing far fewer nutrients than what you have eaten. And here is why. The food you consume gets processed in the intestines. There, along with the digestive juices from the pancreas and liver, the intestine muscles 'churn' the food so it is broken down, the nutrients safely distributed throughout the body and then eliminated. But, when the intestines are inflamed, their muscles do a poor job of processing the food, which means that the food will not get broken down as it should. It will not move out of the body along with many of the unprocessed nutrients that you consumed, but are unable to retain. That is why taking some supplements may be the smart choice for you. However, I strongly suggest you consult with your doctor before buying any over-the-counter multivitamins.

The 6-Week Meal Plan

Below, you will find a well-planned 6-week low fiber meal plan that will get you started and give you a pretty good idea of how to cook using low fiber ingredients. But before you put you put your apron on and start cooking, know that this is just a general meal plan. The low fiber diet is, in fact, a very individualized diet, so keep in mind that you will probably have to go with trial and error in order to tailor the meal plan according to your specific needs.

In case you are wondering why 6 weeks, it is because most people are advised to follow a low fiber diet for 6 weeks. It also takes approximately 6 weeks for your bowels to start function normally following surgery, so I thought that a 6-week meal plan would be the perfect choice — in order to give most of you something tangible to work with.

If you find that a certain dish or ingredient in this meal plan upsets your stomach, try to cook it — if you typically eat it raw. If not, choose a low-fat or low-dairy option. If that still doesn't work for you, then it is probably best to omit that type of food. Remember that we are all unique and that our bowels work differently.

WEEK 1

Day 1:

Breakfast:

- 1 piece of White Bread

- 1 tsp Butter

- 1 tbsp Seedless Fruit Jam

- ½ cup Milk

Snack 1:

- ½ Cucumber

- 2 tbsp Cream Cheese

Lunch:

- 1 cup Cream of Chicken Soup (made with allowed ingredients)

- 2 tbsp Croutons (softened in the soup)

Snack 2:

- 1 ripe Banana

Dinner:

- 4-ounce Salmon Fillet

- ½ cup cooked Veggies

- ½ cup cooked White Rice

Day 2:

Breakfast:

-       1 hard-boiled Egg

-       1 piece of White Bread

-       1 ounce Cheese of choice

-       ½ peeled and deseeded Tomato

Snack 1:

-       4 Plain Biscuits

-       1 cup of Milk

Lunch:

-       ½ cup cooked Rice

-       ½ cup chopped Lettuce

-       ½ Cucumber

-       3 ounces shredded cooked Chicken

-       1 tbsp Mild Salad Dressing

Snack 2:

-       ½ cup Melon Chunks

-       ½ cup Fruit Juice, without pulp

Dinner:

- 4 ounces well-cooked White Pasta

- 2 tbsp homemade Tomato Sauce, without seeds and skin

- 3 ounces well-cooked ground Beef

Day 3:

Breakfast:

- ¾ cup Cornflakes

- 1 cup Milk

- ½ Banana

Snack 1:

- 1 cooked Carrot

- ¼ Cucumber

- 2 tbsp Cream Cheese

Lunch:

- 1 cup Veggie Noodle Soup

- ½ slice of Bread

- 1 small Peach

Snack 2:

- ½ cup Rice Pudding

Dinner:

-   1 serving Mashed Potatoes

-   1 well-cooked Chicken Breast

-   4 well-cooked Asparagus Spears

Day 4:

Breakfast:

-   1 scrambled Egg

-   1 piece of Bread

-   1 tsp Butter

-   1 ounce Cheese

-   ½ cup Milk

Snack 1:

-   1 scoop Vanilla Ice Cream

-   3 Graham Crackers

Lunch:

-   ½ cup Veggie Broth

-   ½ small cooked Zucchini

-   2 ounces cooked Mushrooms

- ½ cup canned Fruit

Snack 2:

- 2 Plain Cookies

- 1 tbsp Seedless Fruit Jam

Dinner:

- 1 serving Lamb stew (made with allowed ingredients)

- ½ slice of White Bread

- 1 cup Veggie Juice, without the pulp

Day 5:

Breakfast:

- ½ White Bagel

- 1 tbsp Cream Cheese

- 1 slice of Bacon

- ½ cup Fruit Juice

Snack 1:

- ½ cup Seedless Grapes

- 2 Crackers

- 1 ounce Cheese

Lunch:

- ½ cup Chicken Broth

- ½ cup cooked White Rice

- 3 ounces well-cooked Fish Fillet

Snack 2:

- 1 cup Yogurt

- 2 tbsp Graham Cracker Crumbs

- ¼ cup Pineapple Chunks

Dinner:

- 1 White Hamburger Bun

- 1 Lettuce Leaf

- 2 Tomato Slices, no skin or seeds

- 3 ounces well-cooked ground Beef Patty

Day 6:

Breakfast:

- ¾ cup Cheerios™

- 1 cup Milk

Snack 1:

- 1 Banana

- 1 tbsp Peanut Butter

Lunch:

- ½ cup Veggie Broth

- 3 ounces well-cooked and shredded Turkey

- ½ cup chopped Lettuce

- ½ cup cooked allowed Veggies

- 1/3 cup cooked White Rice

Snack 2:

- 1 Plain Muffin

- ½ cup Milk

Dinner:

- 1 Green Bell Pepper stuffed with 2 tbsp cooked White Rice, 2 tbsp well-cooked ground Beef, and baked

- ½ Tomato

- ¼ Cucumber

- 1 scoop of Ice Cream

Day 7:

Breakfast:

-   2 small White Pancakes

-   2 tbsp Whipped Cream

-   2 tbsp pureed allowed Fruit

-   1 cup Milk

Snack 1:

-   ¾ cup Pudding of choice

Lunch:

-   Peanut Butter and Jelly Sandwich

-   1 cup Fruit Juice, without pulp

Snack 2:

-   5 Crackers

-   2 tbsp Cream Cheese

-   1 cooked Carrot

Dinner:

-   1 small can Tuna in water

-   4 ounces White Pasta

-   1 tbsp Mayonnaise

-   1 tbsp grated Parmesan Cheese

-   1/3 cup canned Apricots

WEEK 2

Day 1

Breakfast:

- 1 scrambled Egg

- 1 slice of Bacon

- 1 piece of White Bread

- ½ Tomato

- 1 slice of Cheddar Cheese

Snack 1:

- 1 slice of Plain Cake

- 1 cup of Milk

Lunch:

- 1 cup Chicken Noodle Soup

- ½ slice of White Bread

- ½ cup Watermelon Chunks

Snack 2:

- 1 cup Sherbet

Dinner:

- 1 cup cooked allowed Veggies

- 4 ounces well-cooked and shredded Turkey

- 1/3 cup cooked White Rice

- 1 cup Fruit Juice, without pulp

Day 2:

Breakfast:

- 2 small White Waffles

- ½ Banana

- 2 tbsp Whipped Cream

- 1 cup Milk

Snack 1:

- 1 cup Fruit chunks of choice

Lunch:

- 1 slice of White Bread

- 1 tbsp Cream Cheese

- 3 ounces well-cooked Fish

- ¼ Cucumber

- ½ Tomato

Snack 2:

- 2 scoops of Favorite Ice Cream

-       2 tbsp Graham Cracker Crumbs

Dinner:

-       1 serving of Beef Stew

-       ½ slice of Bread

-       ½ cup Salad of choice, with allowed ingredients

-       ½ cup seedless Grapes

Day 3:

Breakfast:

-       1 slice of Bread

-       2 tsp Butter

-       1 tbsp Seedless Fruit Jam

-       1 cup Milk

Snack 1:

-       ¾ cup Rice Pudding

Lunch:

-       ½ cup Chicken Broth

-       ½ cup chopped Lettuce

-       1 small can Tuna in water

- ¼ Cucumber

- 1 tbsp Mayonnaise

- ½ Tomato

- 1 tsp grated Parmesan Cheese

Snack 2:

- ½ cup Yogurt

- ¾ cup Watermelon Chunks

Dinner:

- ½ White Hamburger Bun

- 4 ounces well-cooked Chicken Breast

- 1 cup Salad of choice, with allowed ingredients

- 1 cup Fruit Juice, without pulp

Day 4:

Breakfast:

- 1 Breakfast Roll

- 1 tbsp Seedless Fruit Jam

- 1 cup Milk

Snack 1:

-    2 ounces Cheese

-    ½ cup seedless Grapes

Lunch:

-    3 ounces well-cooked Beef Patty

     ½ White Hamburger Bun

-    ½ cup Veggie slices of choice, allowed ingredients only

Snack 2:

-    1 slice Peach Cobbler

-    ½ cup Milk

Dinner:

-    ½ cup Mashed Potatoes

-    4 ounces well-cooked Fish Fillet

-    4 well-cooked Asparagus spears

-    1 well-cooked Carrot

-    1 scoop of Ice Cream

DAY 5:

Breakfast:

-    1 hard-boiled Egg

- ½ White Bagel

- 1 tbsp Cream Cheese

- ½ cup Yogurt

- ½ Tomato

Snack 1:

- ¾ cup Melon Chunks

Lunch:

- ½ cup White Rice

- ½ cup sliced Veggies, allowed ingredients only

- 3 ounces well-cooked and shredded Chicken

- 1 small Peach

Snack 2:

- 3 Plain Cookies

- 1 cup Milk

Dinner:

- 1 cup Fish Stew

- 1 slice of Bread

- ½ cup Salad of choice, with allowed ingredients

- 1 small Fruit of choice

DAY 6:

Breakfast:

-      2 small Pancakes

-      1 tbsp Honey

-      ½ Banana

-      1 cup of Milk

Snack 1:

-      4 Baby Carrots, cooked

-      ¼ Cucumber

-      2 tbsp Cream Cheese

-      2 Crackers

Lunch:

-      1 slice of White Bread

-      1 tbsp Sour Cream

-      3 ounces well-cooked Lean Meat, of choice

-      1 cup Fruit Juice, without pulp

Snack 2:

-      ½ cup Pudding

-      1 Apricot

Dinner:

-     4 ounces White Pasta, cooked

-     2 tbsp favorite Mild Sauce

-     3 ounces well-cooked ground Turkey

-     1 tbsp Parmesan Cheese

-     ½ cup Grape Juice

Day 7:

Breakfast:

-     1 scrambled Egg

-     1 Bacon Slice

-     1 slice of White Bread

-     1 tbsp Cottage Cheese

-     ½ Tomato

-     ½ cup Fruit Juice

Snack 1:

-     2 Vanilla Wafers

-     ½ cup Milk

Lunch:

- 1 cup Chicken Rice Soup

- 1 cup Salad of choice, with allowed ingredients

Snack 2:

- ½ cup canned Fruit

  ¼ cup Yogurt

- 1 tbsp Graham Cracker Crumbs

Dinner:

- 2 small well-cooked ground Lamb Patties

- ½ cup cooked White Rice

- 2 ounces cooked Mushrooms

- 1 well- cooked Carrot

- 1 scoop of Ice Cream

WEEK 3

Day 1:

Breakfast:

- ¾ cup Cornflakes

- 1 cup Milk

Snack 1:

- 1 cup Watermelon Chunks

- 2 ounces Cheese

Lunch:

- 1 cup Clean Veggie Soup

- ½ cup boiled Potato chunks

- 3 ounces well-cooked Fish Fillet

- 1 Apricot

Snack 2:

- 1 slice of Pie, made with white flour and allowed ingredients only

- ½ cup of Milk

Dinner:

- 3 ounces well-cooked and tender Beef

- 1 cup Salad of choice, with allowed ingredients

- 3 ounces cooked Mushrooms

- 4 cooked Baby Carrots

- 1 cup of Fruit Juice, without pulp

Day 2:

Breakfast:

- 1 Breakfast Roll

- 1 tbsp Fruit Jam

- 1 cup of Milk

Snack 1:

- ½ cup Seedless Grapes

- 3 Crackers

- 2 ounces Cheese

Lunch:

- Peanut Butter and Jelly Sandwich

Snack 2:

- 2 tbsp Yogurt

- 1 tbsp Cream Cheese

- 2 tbsp Graham Cracker Crumbs

-       1/3 cup chopped Canned Fruit

Dinner:

-       ½ cup cooked White Rice

-       3 ounces well-cooked tender Meat

-       1 cup Salad, of choice, with allowed ingredients

-       ½ cup Fruit Juice, without pulp

Day 3:

Breakfast:

-       Breakfast smoothie made with ½ cup Yogurt, 1 Banana, 3 tbsp Graham Cracker Crumbs, and ½ Peach

Snack 1:

-       3 Gingersnap Cookies

-       ½ cup of Milk

Lunch:

-       1 cup Cream of Chicken Soup

-       ½ slice of Bread

-       1/3 cup Cantaloupe chunks

Snack 2:

-       1 cup of Jell-O®

Dinner:

-        ½ Zucchini stuffed with 2 tbsp cooked White Rice, 2 tbsp well-cooked ground Meat, and baked

-        ½ cup chopped Lettuce

-        ½ Tomato

-        ½ cup Grape Juice

Day 4:

Breakfast:

-        1 scrambled Egg

-        ½ Tomato

-        ¼ cup shredded and cooked Zucchini

-        2 tbsp Ricotta Cheese

-        1 slice of White Bread

-        ½ cup Fruit Juice, without pulp

Snack 1:

-        1 Banana

-        1 tbsp Creamy Peanut Butter

Lunch:

-        1 cup Rice Salad with allowed veggies

- 3 ounces well-cooked Salmon Fillet

- 1 Apricot

Snack 2:

- 1 slice of Plain Cake

  1 cup of Milk

Dinner:

- 3 ounces well-cooked Lamb

- 2 ounces cooked Mushrooms

- ½ cup boiled Potatoes

- ½ cup Sherbet

Day 5:

Breakfast:

- 1 hard-boiled Egg

- 1 Bacon Slice

- 1 slice of White Bread

- 1 tbsp Cream Cheese

- ¼ Tomato

- ½ cup Yogurt

Snack 1:

-       1 Egg Custard

Lunch:

-       ½ cup Chicken Broth

-       1 slice of Bread

-       3 ounces well-cooked and shredded Chicken

-       1 tbsp Ricotta

Snack 2:

-       ¾ cup Melon Chunks

Dinner:

-       4 ounces cooked White Pasta

-       ½ cup cooked Veggies

-       1 ounce Mozzarella Cheese

-       1 tsp Sour Cream

-       1 cup of Fruit Juice, without pulp

Day 6:

Breakfast:

-       ¾ cup Rice Krispies®

- 1 cup of Milk

Snack 1:

- 1 cup of Pudding

Lunch 1:

- ½ Cucumber

- 1 cooked Carrot

- 2 ounces Cheese

- ½ cup chopped Lettuce

- 1 cup Clean Chicken Soup

Snack 2:

- 3 Plain Cookies

- ½ cup of Milk

Dinner:

- ½ cup mashed Potatoes

- 3 ounces well-cooked ground Meat

- ½ cup cooked Veggies

- 1/3 cup canned Fruit

- 1 scoop of Vanilla Ice Cream

Day 7:

Breakfast:

- ½ Bagel

- 2 Bacon Slices

- 1 tbsp Cream Cheese

- ½ cup Fruit Juice

Snack 1:

- 1 cup cooked mixed Veggies

- 1 ounce Cheese

Lunch:

- ½ cup canned Fruits

- 1 Egg Custard

- ½ cup Milk

Snack 2:

- 1 cup seedless Grapes

Dinner:

- 1 cup of Beef or Lamb Stew

- 1 slice of White Bread

- 1 Apricot

WEEK 4

Day 1:

Breakfast:

- 2 small White Waffles

- 1 tsp Honey

- ½ Banana

- 1 cup of Milk

Snack 1:

- 4 Crackers

- 4 cooked Baby Carrots

- 2 ounces of Cheese

Lunch:

- 1 cup of Creamy Mushroom Soup

- 2 tbsp Croutons, softened in the soup

- 2 ounces canned Pineapple

Snack 2:

- ½ cup Yogurt

- ½ cup canned Fruit

Dinner:

- ½ cup White Rice

- 1 3-ounce well-cooked Beef Patty

- ½ cup cooked Veggies

- 1 scoop of Ice Cream

Day 2:

Breakfast:

- 1 hard-boiled Egg

- 1 piece of White Bread

- 1 tsp Butter

- 2 Cheddar Cheese Slices

- ½ cup Yogurt

Snack 1:

- 1 cup of Watermelon Chunks

Lunch:

- 1 cup of clean Veggie Soup

- 3 ounces of well-cooked Fish

- 3 ounces of cooked White Noodles

Snack 2:

- 3 Plain Cookies

- ½ cup of Milk

Dinner:

- 1 slice of Shepherd's Pie, made with allowed ingredients

- ½ cup canned Fruit

Day 3:

Breakfast:

- ¾ cup Cheerios™

- 1 cup of Milk

Snack 1:

- ½ cup Grapes

- ½ cup Melon Chunks

Lunch:

- 2 White Bread slices

- 2 tsp Sour Cream

- 1 Bacon Slice

- 1 Cheddar Cheese Slice

- 2 Tomato Slices

Snack 2:

-      3/4 cup Rice Pudding

Dinner:

-      ½ cup Mashed Potatoes

-      4 Meatballs

-      2 tbsp Tomato Sauce

-      1 Peach

Day 4:

Breakfast:

-      2 small White Pancakes

-      2 tbsp Applesauce

-      1 tbsp Whipped Cream

-      1 cup of Milk

Snack 1:

-      1 cup of Jell-O®

Lunch:

-      ½ cup of cooked White Rice

-      3 ounces of well-cooked and shredded Chicken Breasts

- 2 tbsp favorite Sauce, made with allowed ingredients

- ½ cup of Fruit Juice, without pulp

Snack 2:

- 1 Banana

- 1 tbsp Creamy Peanut Butter

Dinner:

- 4 ounces well-cooked Salmon Fillet

- 2 ounces of cooked White Pasta

- 4 cooked Asparagus spears

- ½ cup chopped lettuce drizzled with salad dressing

Day 5:

Breakfast:

- 1 slice of White Bread

- 2 tsp Butter

- 1 tbsp Fruit Jam

- 1 cup of Milk

Snack 1:

- 1 Egg Custard

Lunch:

- 1 cup of Creamy Chicken Soup

- 1 slice of White Bread

Snack 2:

- 1 slice of Plain Cake (such as Angel Food Cake)

- ½ cup of Milk

Dinner:

- 1 cup of Rice salad with veggies

- 3 ounces of well-cooked Lamb

- ½ cup of canned Fruit

Day 6:

Breakfast:

- 1 hard-boiled Egg

- ½ Bagel

- 1 slice of Bacon

- 1 tbsp Ricotta Cheese

- ½ cup of Fruit Juice, without the pulp

Snack:

- 1 Tomato

- 2 Mozzarella Slices

Lunch:

- 3-ounces well-cooked Hamburger

Snack 2:

- 4 Plain Cookies

- 1 cup of Milk

Dinner:

- 4 ounces cooked White Pasta

- 3 ounces of well-cooked and cubed Salmon

- 1 tbsp Pasta Sauce

- 1 scoop of Ice Cream

Day 7:

Breakfast:

- 1 Plain Muffin

- ½ Banana

- 1 cup of Milk

Snack 1:

- ½ cup of Yogurt

- 2 tbsp Graham Cracker Crumbs

- 1 Peach

Lunch:

- 1 cup of Clean Soup (any non-creamy vegetable or chicken soup)

- 1 slice of White Bread

- 1 tbsp Cream Cheese

- 1 Bacon Slice

Snack 2:

- 1 cup of Melon Chunks

Dinner:

- 2 ounces cooked Mushrooms

- ½ cup of cooked White Rice

- 3 ounces of well-cooked and tender Steak

- ½ cup of Fruit Juice, without pulp

WEEK 5:

Day 1:

Breakfast:

- 1 Breakfast Pastry, of choice

- 1 cup of Milk

Snack 1:

- ½ cup of canned Fruit

- ½ Banana

Lunch:

- ½ cup of Veggie Broth

- 1 can Tuna in water

- 1 Cucumber

- ½ cup chopped Iceberg Lettuce

- ½ Tomato

- 2 ounces Cheese

Snack 2:

- 1 piece of Peach Cobbler

Dinner:

- 1 cup of Chicken and Mushroom Risotto

- ½ cup Watermelon Chunks

Day 2:

Breakfast:

- 1 slice of Egg Quiche with allowed ingredients

- 1 cup of Fruit Juice

Snack 1:

- 1 Ripe Banana

- 1 tbsp Creamy Peanut Butter

Lunch:

- ½ cup cooked White Rice

- 3 ounces well-cooked and shredded Turkey

- 2 Mozzarella Slices

- ¼ Tomato

Snack 2:

- 1 piece of Plain Cake or 4 plain cookies

- 1 cup of Milk

Dinner:

- 3 ounces well-cooked and pulled Lamb

-      1 White Bun

-      1 Lettuce Leaf

-      2 tsp Mayonnaise

-      4 Cucumber Slices

Day 3:

Breakfast:

-      ¾ cup allowed Cereal

-      1 cup of Milk

Snack 1:

-      4 Graham Crackers

-      1 Peach

Lunch:

-      1 cup of Chicken Noodle Soup

-      1 cup of Salad of choice, with allowed ingredients

Snack 2:

-      1 cup of Frozen Yogurt made with allowed fruit

Dinner:

-      1 cooked Carrot,

- 2 ounces cooked Zucchini

- 1 cooked Green Pepper

- 1 well-cooked Salmon Fillet

- ½ cup Melon chunks

Day 4:

Breakfast:

- 1 scrambled Egg with 2 ounces of cooked Mushrooms

- 1 tbsp Cottage Cheese

- 1 slice of White Bread

- ½ cup of Fruit Juice, without pulp

Snack 1:

- 1 cup of Grapes

- 1 ounce Goat Cheese

Lunch:

- Peanut Butter and Jelly sandwich

Snack 2:

- 1 cup of Pudding

Dinner:

- ½ cup of mashed Potatoes

- 4 ounces well-cooked cubed Chicken Breast

- ¼ Cucumber

- ½ Tomato

  ½ cup chopped Lettuce

- 2 tsp Salad Dressing

- ½ cup Honeydew Chunks

Day 5:

Breakfast:

- ½ Bagel

- 1 tbsp Cream Cheese

- 1 Bacon Slice

- 1 cup of Fruit Juice, without pulp

Snack 1:

- 1 cup of shredded and cooked beets and carrots

- 1 ounce Cheese

Lunch:

- 1 cup of Yogurt

- 3 tbsp Graham Cracker Crumbs

- 1 tsp Honey, optional

- ½ cup canned Fruit

Snack 2:

- 1 small Pastry

Dinner:

- 1 cup of Lamb Stew

- 1 slice of White Bread

- 1 small Peach

Day 6:

Breakfast:

- 1 slice of allowed Frittata

- 1 slice of White Bread

- ½ cup of Grape Juice

Snack 1:

- 1 slice of Peach Pie

- 1 cup of Milk

Lunch:

-     1 cup of Clean Chicken Soup

-     ½ cup Mushroom Risotto

-     1 Apricot

Snack 2:

    ¼ cup Watermelon Chunks

-     2 ounces Cheese

Dinner:

-     3 ounces cooked White Pasta

-     3 ounces well-cooked Beef

-     2 ounces cooked Mushrooms

-     ½ Tomato

-     1 scoop of Ice Cream

Day 7:

Breakfast:

-     2 small Pancakes

-     ½ cup chopped canned Fruit

-     2 tbsp Whipped Cream

-     ½ cup of Milk

Snack 1:

-    4 Crackers

-    ½ Cucumber

-    2 tbsp Cream Cheese

Lunch:

-    Bacon and Cheddar Sandwich

-    ½ cup of Fruit Juice, without pulp

Dinner:

-    1 serving of cooked White Lasagna with ground beef and tomato sauce

-    ½ cup Melon Chunks

WEEK 6

Day 1:

Breakfast:

-       ¾ cup Cornflakes

-       1 cup Milk

Snack 1:

-       1 cup of Jell-O™

Lunch:

-       1 cup of Blended Soup

-       3 ounces well-cooked cubed Salmon

-       3 ounces of cooked Noodles

Snack 2:

-       ½ cup Yogurt

-       ½ cup canned Fruit

Dinner:

-       ½ cup Mashed Potatoes

-       2 small well-cooked ground Beef Patties

-       1 cooked Carrot

-       1 scoop of Ice Cream

Day 2:

Breakfast:

-        1 hard-boiled Egg

-        1 slice of White Bread

-        2 tsp Butter

-        1 ounce Cheese

-        1 cup of Fruit Juice, without pulp

Snack 1:

-        1 Vanilla Muffin

-        ½ cup of Milk

Lunch:

-        1 slice of White Bread

-        1 tbsp Cream Cheese

-        2 Bacon slices

-        1 cup of Salad of choice, with allowed ingredients

Snack 2:

-        ¾ cup of Rice Pudding

Dinner:

- 1 cup of Blended Veggie Soup

- 3 ounces of well-cooked Beef Steak

- ½ cup boiled Potatoes

- 1 Apricot

Day 3:

Breakfast:

- ½ cup Yogurt

- 1 Peach

- 3 tbsp Graham Cracker Crumbs

- ½ Banana

Snack 1:

- 4 Crackers

- 1 ounce Cheese

- ½ cup seedless Grapes

Lunch:

- ½ cup of Veggie Broth

- ½ cup of cooked White Rice

- 3 ounces of well-cooked Turkey

-   ½ cup of chopped Lettuce drizzled with some salad dressing

Snack 2:

-   1 slice of Pie

-   ½ cup of Milk

Dinner:

-   1 serving of Mac and Cheese

Day 4:

Breakfast:

-   2 savory Muffins with Bacon and Cheese

-   1 cup of Fruit Juice, without pulp

Snack 1:

-   ½ cup Watermelon Chunks

-   ½ cup Honeydew Chunks

Lunch:

-   1 cup of creamy Squash soup

-   2 tbsp Croutons, softened in soup

-   1 Apricot

Snack 2:

- 3 Vanilla Wafers

- 1 cup of Milk

Dinner:

- 1 cup Risotto with Mushrooms

  1 tbsp Parmesan Cheese

- ½ cup canned Fruit

Day 5:

Breakfast:

- ¾ cup Special K® Cereal

- 1 cup of Milk

Snack 1:

- 4 Graham Crackers

- 1 Peach

Lunch:

- 1 White Hamburger Bun

- 3 ounces of well-cooked and pulled Lamb

- 2 Tomato Slices

- 1 Lettuce Leaf

- 1 tsp Mayonnaise

Snack 2:

- 1 piece of allowed Pie

- 1/2 cup of Fruit Juice, strained

Dinner:

- 4 ounces cooked White Spaghetti

- 3 ounces well-cooked ground Beef

- 2 tbsp Tomato Sauce

- 2 scoops of Ice Cream of choice

Day 6:

Breakfast:

- 1 Bagel

- 1 hard-boiled Egg

- 2 tbsp Cream Cheese

- 1 Fruit Juice, strained

Snack 1:

- 1 Vanilla Muffin

- ½ cup of Milk

Lunch:

-       1 cup of Fish Stew

-       1 slice of White Bread

-       1 Apricot

Snack 2.

-       1 cup of Pudding

Dinner:

-       1 White Hamburger Bun

-       3 ounces of well-cooked ground Beef Patty

-       2 Cheddar Cheese Slices

-       1 Lettuce Leaf

-       2 Onion rings

-       2 Tomato slices

Day 7:

Breakfast:

-       2 scrambled Eggs

-       1 tbsp Cottage Cheese

-       1 piece of toasted White Bread

-     2 tsp Butter

-     1 cup of Fruit Juice, strained

Snack 1:

-     1 cup Watermelon Chunks

Lunch:

-     1 cup of Chicken Noodle Soup

-     1 cup of Salad of choice, with allowed ingredients

-     1 Peach

Snack 2:

-     1 piece of Plain Cake

-     1 cup of Milk

Dinner:

-     1 serving of Pot Roast (lamb or beef) with some cooked carrots and potatoes on the side

-     2 scoops of Ice Cream of choice

Conclusion

Now that you know what you have to do in order to restore balance to your bowels, the next step is to simply take advantage of the advice found in this book, and start your healing process today.

I have really done my best to include all of the important information that can help a person with compromised bowel health improve digestion and increase dietary tolerance.

Win a free

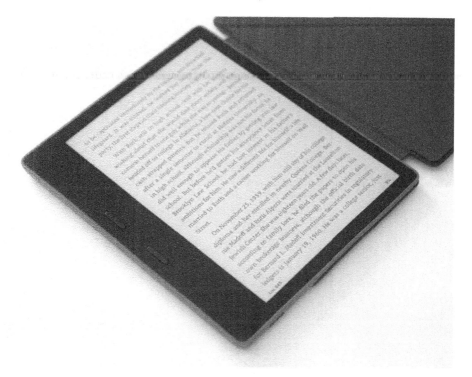

kindle
OASIS

Let us know what you thought of this book to enter the sweepstake at:

booksfor.review/lowfiber

Made in the USA
Coppell, TX
08 April 2021